Lose Weight with Infused Water

Diet Journal

Track Your Journey to Optimum Health

Emily R. Stone

Publisher's Notes

This publication is intended to provide helpful and informative information. It is not intended to diagnose, treat, cure, or prevent any health problem or condition, nor is intended to replace the advice of a physician. No action should be taken solely on the contents of this book. Always consult your physician or qualified health-care professional on any matters regarding your health and before adopting any suggestions in this book or drawing inferences from it.

The author and publisher specifically disclaim all responsibility for any liability, loss or risk, personal or otherwise, which is incurred as a consequence, directly or indirectly, from the use or application of any contents of this book.

Diet Journal Edition 1

ISBN: 9781634289672

Printed in the United States of America.

How to Use This Journal

Use this great ***Diet Journal*** to track your journey to optimum health and weight loss. Record what you eat and the infused water recipes you drink on a daily basis. Having a written record of what and when you eat can be a helpful tool in achieving your goals. Once you start to lose weight and improve your overall health, record everything and make detailed notes. If you ever feel yourself starting to slip back into old eating habits, you can easily replicate your previous successes by referring back to this journal.

It is also designed to help you identify which infused water recipes are the most effective for your overall health and diet needs. Whether your goal is to increase immunity, energy levels, or metabolism, keeping track of the water you drink, and the times you drink it makes it easy to learn what works best for your body.

About the Author

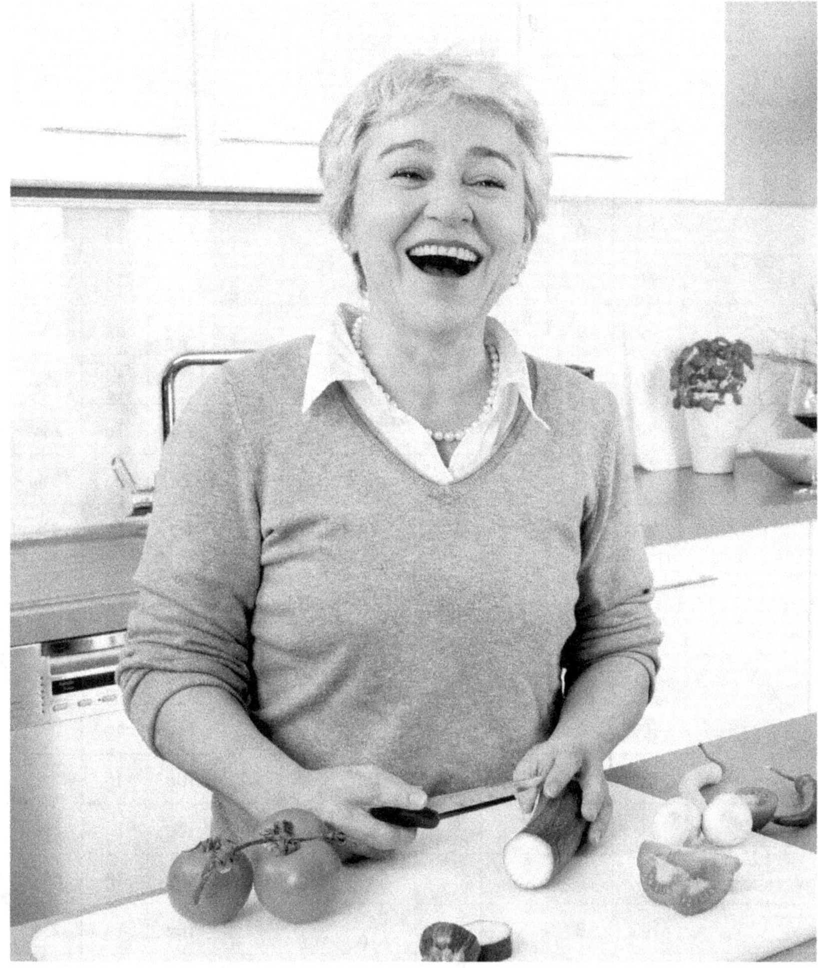

Emily R. Stone loves to eat, but she doesn't like putting on extra pounds. When researching her popular book, ***Mediterranean Diet: 50 of the Best Mediterranean Diet Recipes for Weight Loss***, Emily discovered that the main key to great health and effortless weight loss was fresh fruits, vegetables and herbs. The results she experienced after switching to a Mediterranean-style diet were nothing short of amazing. She felt great, had energy throughout the day, slept better at night, and - best of all - stopped gaining weight!

To complement her healthy Mediterranean eating style, Emily started drinking infused water. The concept of infused water, and learning which fruits, vegetables and herbs went well together, turned out to be a wonderful adventure of discovery. Not only did her infused-water creations taste delicious, helping Emily to drink more water throughout the day, but they provided much-needed vitamins and nutrients. ***Lose Weight with Infused Water: Recipes for Optimum Health*** features her favorite infused-water recipes.

Ms. Stone loves sharing her knowledge and experience with others who may be searching for ways to improve their health, feel better, and lose weight. She recorded her success in a custom diet journal she created on her computer. This is an exact replica of Emily's journal. Now you can track your progress just as she did to lose weight, drink more water, and improve your overall health with the ***Infused Water to Lose Weight Diet Journal***!

Raw, edible weight portion.
Percent Daily Values (%DV) are
based on a 2,000 calorie diet.

Fruits / Serving Size (gram weight/ounce weight)	Calories	Calories from Fat	Total Fat (g)	Total Fat %DV	Sodium (mg)	Sodium %DV	Potassium (mg)	Potassium %DV	Total Carbohydrate (g)	Total Carbohydrate %DV	Dietary Fiber (g)	Dietary Fiber %DV	Sugars (g)	Protein (g)	Vitamin A %DV	Vitamin C %DV	Calcium %DV	Iron %DV
Apple — 1 large (242 g/8 oz)	130	0	0	0	0	0	260	7	34	11	5	20	25g	1g	2%	8%	2%	2%
Avocado — California, 1/5 medium (30 g/1.1 oz)	50	35	4.5	7	0	0	140	4	3	1	1	4	0g	1g	0%	4%	0%	2%
Banana — 1 medium (126 g/4.5 oz)	110	0	0	0	0	0	450	13	30	10	3	12	19g	1g	2%	15%	0%	2%
Cantaloupe — 1/4 medium (134 g/4.8 oz)	50	0	0	0	20	1	240	7	12	4	1	4	11g	1g	120%	80%	2%	2%
Grapefruit — 1/2 medium (154 g/5.5 oz)	60	0	0	0	0	0	160	5	15	5	2	8	11g	1g	35%	100%	4%	0%
Grapes — 3/4 cup (126 g/4.5 oz)	90	0	0	0	15	1	240	7	23	8	1	4	20g	0g	0%	2%	2%	0%
Honeydew Melon — 1/10 medium melon (134 g/4.8 oz)	50	0	0	0	30	1	210	6	12	4	1	4	11g	1g	2%	45%	2%	2%
Kiwifruit — 2 medium (148 g/5.3 oz)	90	10	1	2	0	0	450	13	20	7	4	16	13g	1g	2%	240%	4%	2%
Lemon — 1 medium (58 g/2.1 oz)	15	0	0	0	0	0	75	2	5	2	2	8	2g	0g	0%	40%	2%	0%
Lime — 1 medium (67 g/2.4 oz)	20	0	0	0	0	0	75	2	7	2	2	8	0g	0g	0%	35%	0%	0%
Nectarine — 1 medium (140 g/5.0 oz)	60	5	0.5	1	0	0	250	7	15	5	2	8	11g	1g	8%	15%	0%	2%
Orange — 1 medium (154 g/5.5 oz)	80	0	0	0	0	0	250	7	19	6	3	12	14g	1g	2%	130%	6%	0%
Peach — 1 medium (147 g/5.3 oz)	60	0	0.5	1	0	0	230	7	15	5	2	8	13g	1g	6%	15%	0%	2%
Pear — 1 medium (166 g/5.9 oz)	100	0	0	0	0	0	190	5	26	9	6	24	16g	1g	0%	10%	2%	0%
Pineapple — 2 slices, 3" diameter, 3/4" thick (112 g/4 oz)	50	0	0	0	10	0	120	3	13	4	1	4	10g	1g	2%	50%	2%	2%
Plums — 2 plums (151 g/5.4 oz)	70	0	0	0	0	0	230	7	19	6	2	8	16g	1g	8%	10%	0%	2%
Strawberries — 8 medium (147g/5.3 oz)	50	0	0	0	0	0	170	5	11	4	2	8	8g	1g	0%	160%	2%	2%
Sweet Cherries — 21 cherries; 1 cup (140 g/5.0 oz)	100	0	0	0	0	0	350	10	26	9	1	4	16g	1g	2%	15%	2%	2%
Tangerine — 1 medium (109 g/3.9 oz)	50	0	0	0	0	0	160	5	13	4	2	8	9g	1g	6%	45%	4%	0%
Watermelon — 1/18 medium melon; 2 cups diced pieces (280 g/10.0 oz)	80	0	0	0	0	0	270	8	21	7	1	4	20g	1g	30%	25%	2%	4%

Raw, edible weight portion.
Percent Daily Values (%DV) are
based on a 2,000 calorie diet.

Vegetables Serving Size (gram weight/ounce weight)	Calories	Calories from Fat	Total Fat g / %DV	Sodium mg / %DV	Potassium mg / %DV	Total Carbohydrate g / %DV	Dietary Fiber g / %DV	Sugars g	Protein g	Vitamin A %DV	Vitamin C %DV	Calcium %DV	Iron %DV
Asparagus 5 spears (93 g/3.3 oz)	20	0	0 / 0	0 / 0	230 / 7	4 / 1	2 / 8	2g	2g	10%	15%	2%	2%
Bell Pepper 1 medium (148 g/5.3 oz)	25	0	0 / 0	40 / 2	220 / 6	6 / 2	2 / 8	4g	1g	4%	190%	2%	4%
Broccoli 1 medium stalk (148 g/5.3 oz)	45	0	0.5 / 1	80 / 3	460 / 13	8 / 3	3 / 12	2g	4g	6%	220%	6%	6%
Carrot 1 carrot, 7" long, 1 1/4" diameter (78 g/2.8 oz)	30	0	0 / 0	60 / 3	250 / 7	7 / 2	2 / 8	5g	1g	110%	10%	2%	2%
Cauliflower 1/6 medium head (99 g/3.5 oz)	25	0	0 / 0	30 / 1	270 / 8	5 / 2	2 / 8	2g	2g	0%	100%	2%	2%
Celery 2 medium stalks (110 g/3.9 oz)	15	0	0 / 0	115 / 5	260 / 7	4 / 1	2 / 8	2g	0g	10%	15%	4%	2%
Cucumber 1/3 medium (99 g/3.5 oz)	10	0	0 / 0	0 / 0	140 / 4	2 / 1	1 / 4	1g	1g	4%	10%	2%	2%
Green (Snap) Beans 3/4 cup cut (83 g/3.0 oz)	20	0	0 / 0	0 / 0	200 / 6	5 / 2	3 / 12	2g	1g	4%	10%	4%	2%
Green Cabbage 1/12 medium head (84 g/3.0 oz)	25	0	0 / 0	20 / 1	190 / 5	5 / 2	2 / 8	3g	1g	0%	70%	4%	2%
Green Onion 1/4 cup chopped (25 g/0.9 oz)	10	0	0 / 0	10 / 0	70 / 2	2 / 1	1 / 4	1g	0g	2%	8%	2%	2%
Iceberg Lettuce 1/6 medium head (89 g/3.2 oz)	10	0	0 / 0	10 / 0	125 / 4	2 / 1	1 / 4	2g	1g	6%	6%	2%	2%
Leaf Lettuce 1 1/2 cups shredded (85 g/3.0 oz)	15	0	0 / 0	35 / 1	170 / 5	2 / 1	1 / 4	1g	1g	130%	6%	2%	4%
Mushrooms 5 medium (84 g/3.0 oz)	20	0	0 / 0	15 / 0	300 / 9	3 / 1	1 / 4	0g	3g	0%	2%	0%	2%
Onion 1 medium (148 g/5.3 oz)	45	0	0 / 0	5 / 0	190 / 5	11 / 4	3 / 12	9g	1g	0%	20%	4%	4%
Potato 1 medium (148 g/5.3 oz)	110	0	0 / 0	0 / 0	620 / 18	26 / 9	2 / 8	1g	3g	0%	45%	2%	6%
Radishes 7 radishes (85 g/3.0 oz)	10	0	0 / 0	55 / 2	190 / 5	3 / 1	1 / 4	2g	0g	0%	30%	2%	2%
Summer Squash 1/2 medium (98 g/3.5 oz)	20	0	0 / 0	0 / 0	260 / 7	4 / 1	2 / 8	2g	1g	6%	30%	2%	2%
Sweet Corn kernels from 1 medium ear (90 g/3.2 oz)	90	20	2.5 / 4	0 / 0	250 / 7	18 / 6	2 / 8	5g	4g	2%	10%	0%	2%
Sweet Potato 1 medium, 5" long, 2"diameter (130 g/4.6 oz)	100	0	0 / 0	70 / 3	440 / 13	23 / 8	4 / 16	7g	2g	120%	30%	4%	4%
Tomato 1 medium (148 g/5.3 oz)	25	0	0 / 0	20 / 1	340 / 10	5 / 2	1 / 4	3g	1g	20%	40%	2%	4%

DATE: _________________________________   WEIGHT: _________________________________

WATER INTAKE: _____________________   INFUSED WATER: _____________________

DAILY GOAL: ____

Increase Immunity   Increase Energy   Detoxification   Increase Metabolism

BREAKFAST

Food	Time	Amount	Calories

Mood: _____________________   Energy: _____________________   Total Calories: _____________________

LUNCH

Food	Time	Amount	Calories

Mood: _____________________   Energy: _____________________   Total Calories: _____________________

DINNER

Food	Time	Amount	Calories

Mood: _____________________   Energy: _____________________   Total Calories: _____________________

SNACKS

Food	Time	Amount	Calories

Mood: _____________   Energy: _____________   Total Calories: _____________

INFUSED WATER

Ingredients	Time	Amount	Mood After

EXERCISE

Activity	Time	Amount	Mood After

NOTES

DATE: _________________________   WEIGHT: _________________________

WATER INTAKE: _________________   INFUSED WATER: _________________

DAILY GOAL: ____

Increase Immunity   Increase Energy   Detoxification   Increase Metabolism

BREAKFAST

Food	Time	Amount	Calories

Mood: _________________   Energy: _________________   Total Calories: _________________

LUNCH

Food	Time	Amount	Calories

Mood: _________________   Energy: _________________   Total Calories: _________________

DINNER

Food	Time	Amount	Calories

Mood: _________________   Energy: _________________   Total Calories: _________________

Food	Time	Amount	Calories

Mood: _________________ Energy: _________________ Total Calories: _________________

INFUSED WATER

Ingredients	Time	Amount	Mood After

EXERCISE

Activity	Time	Amount	Mood After

NOTES

DATE: ___________________________ WEIGHT: ___________________________

WATER INTAKE: _____________________ INFUSED WATER: ___________________

DAILY GOAL: ____

Increase Immunity   Increase Energy   Detoxification   Increase Metabolism

BREAKFAST				
Food		Time	Amount	Calories
Mood: _____________	Energy: _____________	Total Calories: _____________		

LUNCH				
Food		Time	Amount	Calories
Mood: _____________	Energy: _____________	Total Calories: _____________		

DINNER				
Food		Time	Amount	Calories
Mood: _____________	Energy: _____________	Total Calories: _____________		

SNACKS

Food	Time	Amount	Calories

Mood: _________________ Energy: _________________ Total Calories: _________________

INFUSED WATER

Ingredients	Time	Amount	Mood After

EXERCISE

Activity	Time	Amount	Mood After

NOTES

DATE: ___________________________   WEIGHT: ___________________________

WATER INTAKE: ___________________   INFUSED WATER: ___________________

DAILY GOAL: ____

Increase Immunity   Increase Energy   Detoxification   Increase Metabolism

BREAKFAST

Food	Time	Amount	Calories

Mood: ________________   Energy: ________________   Total Calories: ________________

LUNCH

Food	Time	Amount	Calories

Mood: ________________   Energy: ________________   Total Calories: ________________

DINNER

Food	Time	Amount	Calories

Mood: ________________   Energy: ________________   Total Calories: ________________

Food		Time	Amount	Calories

Mood: _________________ Energy: _________________ Total Calories: _________________

INFUSED WATER

Ingredients	Time	Amount	Mood After

EXERCISE

Activity	Time	Amount	Mood After

NOTES

DATE: _______________________________   WEIGHT: ______________________________

WATER INTAKE: ___________________   INFUSED WATER: ___________________

DAILY GOAL: ____

Increase Immunity   Increase Energy   Detoxification   Increase Metabolism

BREAKFAST

Food		Time	Amount	Calories
Mood: _______________	Energy: _______________	Total Calories: _______________		

LUNCH

Food		Time	Amount	Calories
Mood: _______________	Energy: _______________	Total Calories: _______________		

DINNER

Food		Time	Amount	Calories
Mood: _______________	Energy: _______________	Total Calories: _______________		

SNACKS

Food	Time	Amount	Calories

Mood: _________________   Energy: _________________   Total Calories: _________________

INFUSED WATER

Ingredients	Time	Amount	Mood After

EXERCISE

Activity	Time	Amount	Mood After

NOTES

DATE: _________________________________   WEIGHT: _________________________________

WATER INTAKE: _____________________   INFUSED WATER: _____________________

DAILY GOAL: ____

Increase Immunity   Increase Energy   Detoxification   Increase Metabolism

BREAKFAST

Food	Time	Amount	Calories

Mood: __________________   Energy: __________________   Total Calories: __________________

LUNCH

Food	Time	Amount	Calories

Mood: __________________   Energy: __________________   Total Calories: __________________

DINNER

Food	Time	Amount	Calories

Mood: __________________   Energy: __________________   Total Calories: __________________

SNACKS

Food	Time	Amount	Calories

Mood: _________________ Energy: _________________ Total Calories: _________________

INFUSED WATER

Ingredients	Time	Amount	Mood After

EXERCISE

Activity	Time	Amount	Mood After

NOTES

DATE: ____________________________   WEIGHT: ____________________________

WATER INTAKE: ____________________   INFUSED WATER: ____________________

DAILY GOAL: ____

Increase Immunity   Increase Energy   Detoxification   Increase Metabolism

BREAKFAST

Food	Time	Amount	Calories

Mood: __________________   Energy: __________________   Total Calories: __________________

LUNCH

Food	Time	Amount	Calories

Mood: __________________   Energy: __________________   Total Calories: __________________

DINNER

Food	Time	Amount	Calories

Mood: __________________   Energy: __________________   Total Calories: __________________

Food	Time	Amount	Calories

Mood: _________________ Energy: _________________ Total Calories: _______________

INFUSED WATER

Ingredients	Time	Amount	Mood After

EXERCISE

Activity	Time	Amount	Mood After

NOTES

DATE: _______________________________   WEIGHT: _______________________________

WATER INTAKE: _____________________   INFUSED WATER: _____________________

DAILY GOAL: ____

Increase Immunity   Increase Energy   Detoxification   Increase Metabolism

BREAKFAST

Food	Time	Amount	Calories

Mood: _________________ Energy: _________________ Total Calories: _________________

LUNCH

Food	Time	Amount	Calories

Mood: _________________ Energy: _________________ Total Calories: _________________

DINNER

Food	Time	Amount	Calories

Mood: _________________ Energy: _________________ Total Calories: _________________

SNACKS

Food	Time	Amount	Calories

Mood: _____________________ Energy: _____________________ Total Calories: _____________________

INFUSED WATER

Ingredients	Time	Amount	Mood After

EXERCISE

Activity	Time	Amount	Mood After

NOTES

DATE: _________________________________   WEIGHT: _____________________________

WATER INTAKE: _____________________   INFUSED WATER: ___________________

DAILY GOAL: ____

Increase Immunity   Increase Energy   Detoxification   Increase Metabolism

BREAKFAST

Food	Time	Amount	Calories

Mood: _________________   Energy: _________________   Total Calories: _______________

LUNCH

Food	Time	Amount	Calories

Mood: _________________   Energy: _________________   Total Calories: _______________

DINNER

Food	Time	Amount	Calories

Mood: _________________   Energy: _________________   Total Calories: _______________

SNACKS

Food	Time	Amount	Calories

Mood: _________________ | Energy: _________________ | Total Calories: _______________

INFUSED WATER

Ingredients	Time	Amount	Mood After

EXERCISE

Activity	Time	Amount	Mood After

NOTES

DATE: ___________________________ WEIGHT: ___________________________

WATER INTAKE: ___________________ INFUSED WATER: ___________________

DAILY GOAL: ____

Increase Immunity   Increase Energy   Detoxification   Increase Metabolism

BREAKFAST

Food		Time	Amount	Calories

Mood: ________________ Energy: ________________ Total Calories: ________________

LUNCH

Food		Time	Amount	Calories

Mood: ________________ Energy: ________________ Total Calories: ________________

DINNER

Food		Time	Amount	Calories

Mood: ________________ Energy: ________________ Total Calories: ________________

SNACKS

Food	Time	Amount	Calories

Mood: _____________________ Energy: _____________________ Total Calories: _____________________

INFUSED WATER

Ingredients	Time	Amount	Mood After

EXERCISE

Activity	Time	Amount	Mood After

NOTES

DATE: _______________________________   WEIGHT: _______________________________

WATER INTAKE: _______________________   INFUSED WATER: _______________________

DAILY GOAL: ____

Increase Immunity   Increase Energy   Detoxification   Increase Metabolism

BREAKFAST

Food	Time	Amount	Calories

Mood: _________________   Energy: _________________   Total Calories: _________________

LUNCH

Food	Time	Amount	Calories

Mood: _________________   Energy: _________________   Total Calories: _________________

DINNER

Food	Time	Amount	Calories

Mood: _________________   Energy: _________________   Total Calories: _________________

Food	Time	Amount	Calories

Mood: _____________________ Energy: _____________________ Total Calories: _____________________

Ingredients	Time	Amount	Mood After

Activity	Time	Amount	Mood After

DATE: _______________________________   WEIGHT: _______________________________

WATER INTAKE: _____________________   INFUSED WATER: _________________________

DAILY GOAL: ____

Increase Immunity   Increase Energy   Detoxification   Increase Metabolism

BREAKFAST

Food	Time	Amount	Calories

Mood: _________________   Energy: _________________   Total Calories: _________________

LUNCH

Food	Time	Amount	Calories

Mood: _________________   Energy: _________________   Total Calories: _________________

DINNER

Food	Time	Amount	Calories

Mood: _________________   Energy: _________________   Total Calories: _________________

SNACKS

Food	Time	Amount	Calories

Mood: _________________   Energy: _________________   Total Calories: _________________

INFUSED WATER

Ingredients	Time	Amount	Mood After

EXERCISE

Activity	Time	Amount	Mood After

NOTES

DATE: ______________________________   WEIGHT: ______________________________

WATER INTAKE: ____________________   INFUSED WATER: ____________________

DAILY GOAL: ____

Increase Immunity   Increase Energy   Detoxification   Increase Metabolism

BREAKFAST

Food	Time	Amount	Calories

Mood: _________________   Energy: _________________   Total Calories: _________________

LUNCH

Food	Time	Amount	Calories

Mood: _________________   Energy: _________________   Total Calories: _________________

DINNER

Food	Time	Amount	Calories

Mood: _________________   Energy: _________________   Total Calories: _________________

SNACKS

Food	Time	Amount	Calories

Mood: _____________________ Energy: _____________________ Total Calories: _____________________

INFUSED WATER

Ingredients	Time	Amount	Mood After

EXERCISE

Activity	Time	Amount	Mood After

NOTES

DATE: _______________________________ WEIGHT: _______________________________

WATER INTAKE: _____________________ INFUSED WATER: _____________________

DAILY GOAL: ____

Increase Immunity   Increase Energy   Detoxification   Increase Metabolism

BREAKFAST

Food	Time	Amount	Calories

Mood: _______________ Energy: _______________ Total Calories: _______________

LUNCH

Food	Time	Amount	Calories

Mood: _______________ Energy: _______________ Total Calories: _______________

DINNER

Food	Time	Amount	Calories

Mood: _______________ Energy: _______________ Total Calories: _______________

Food		Time	Amount	Calories

Mood: ______________________ Energy: ______________________ Total Calories: ______________________

INFUSED WATER

Ingredients	Time	Amount	Mood After

EXERCISE

Activity	Time	Amount	Mood After

NOTES

DATE: _______________________________ WEIGHT: _______________________________

WATER INTAKE: _______________________ INFUSED WATER: ____________________

DAILY GOAL: ____

Increase Immunity   Increase Energy   Detoxification   Increase Metabolism

BREAKFAST

Food	Time	Amount	Calories

Mood: ___________________ Energy: ___________________ Total Calories: ___________________

LUNCH

Food	Time	Amount	Calories

Mood: ___________________ Energy: ___________________ Total Calories: ___________________

DINNER

Food	Time	Amount	Calories

Mood: ___________________ Energy: ___________________ Total Calories: ___________________

SNACKS

Food	Time	Amount	Calories

Mood: _____________________ Energy: _____________________ Total Calories: _______________

INFUSED WATER

Ingredients	Time	Amount	Mood After

EXERCISE

Activity	Time	Amount	Mood After

NOTES

DATE: _________________________________ WEIGHT: _________________________________

WATER INTAKE: _____________________ INFUSED WATER: _____________________

DAILY GOAL: ____

Increase Immunity   Increase Energy   Detoxification   Increase Metabolism

BREAKFAST

Food	Time	Amount	Calories

Mood: _______________ Energy: _______________ Total Calories: _______________

LUNCH

Food	Time	Amount	Calories

Mood: _______________ Energy: _______________ Total Calories: _______________

DINNER

Food	Time	Amount	Calories

Mood: _______________ Energy: _______________ Total Calories: _______________

SNACKS

Food	Time	Amount	Calories

Mood: _________________   Energy: _________________   Total Calories: _________________

INFUSED WATER

Ingredients	Time	Amount	Mood After

EXERCISE

Activity	Time	Amount	Mood After

NOTES

DATE: _________________________   WEIGHT: _____________________

WATER INTAKE: __________________   INFUSED WATER: _______________

DAILY GOAL: ____

Increase Immunity   Increase Energy   Detoxification   Increase Metabolism

BREAKFAST

Food	Time	Amount	Calories

Mood: _______________   Energy: _______________   Total Calories: _______________

LUNCH

Food	Time	Amount	Calories

Mood: _______________   Energy: _______________   Total Calories: _______________

DINNER

Food	Time	Amount	Calories

Mood: _______________   Energy: _______________   Total Calories: _______________

SNACKS

Food	Time	Amount	Calories

Mood: ___________________   Energy: ___________________   Total Calories: ___________________

INFUSED WATER

Ingredients	Time	Amount	Mood After

EXERCISE

Activity	Time	Amount	Mood After

NOTES

DATE: _________________________   WEIGHT: _________________________

WATER INTAKE: _________________   INFUSED WATER: _________________

DAILY GOAL: ____

Increase Immunity   Increase Energy   Detoxification   Increase Metabolism

BREAKFAST

Food	Time	Amount	Calories

Mood: _________________ Energy: _________________ Total Calories: _________________

LUNCH

Food	Time	Amount	Calories

Mood: _________________ Energy: _________________ Total Calories: _________________

DINNER

Food	Time	Amount	Calories

Mood: _________________ Energy: _________________ Total Calories: _________________

Food	Time	Amount	Calories

Mood: _____________________ Energy: _____________________ Total Calories: _____________________

INFUSED WATER

Ingredients	Time	Amount	Mood After

EXERCISE

Activity	Time	Amount	Mood After

NOTES

DATE: _______________________________   WEIGHT: _______________________________

WATER INTAKE: _______________________   INFUSED WATER: _____________________

DAILY GOAL: ____

Increase Immunity   Increase Energy   Detoxification   Increase Metabolism

BREAKFAST

Food	Time	Amount	Calories

Mood: ________________   Energy: ________________   Total Calories: ________________

LUNCH

Food	Time	Amount	Calories

Mood: ________________   Energy: ________________   Total Calories: ________________

DINNER

Food	Time	Amount	Calories

Mood: ________________   Energy: ________________   Total Calories: ________________

SNACKS

Food	Time	Amount	Calories

Mood: ___________________   Energy: ___________________   Total Calories: ___________________

INFUSED WATER

Ingredients	Time	Amount	Mood After

EXERCISE

Activity	Time	Amount	Mood After

NOTES

DATE: ___________________________   WEIGHT: ___________________________

WATER INTAKE: _________________   INFUSED WATER: _________________

DAILY GOAL: ____

Increase Immunity   Increase Energy   Detoxification   Increase Metabolism

BREAKFAST

Food		Time	Amount	Calories
Mood: _____________	Energy: _____________	Total Calories: _____________		

LUNCH

Food		Time	Amount	Calories
Mood: _____________	Energy: _____________	Total Calories: _____________		

DINNER

Food		Time	Amount	Calories
Mood: _____________	Energy: _____________	Total Calories: _____________		

Food	Time	Amount	Calories

Mood: _____________________ Energy: _____________________ Total Calories: _____________________

INFUSED WATER

Ingredients	Time	Amount	Mood After

EXERCISE

Activity	Time	Amount	Mood After

NOTES

DATE: _______________________   WEIGHT: _____________________

WATER INTAKE: _________________   INFUSED WATER: ______________

DAILY GOAL: ____

Increase Immunity   Increase Energy   Detoxification   Increase Metabolism

BREAKFAST				
Food		Time	Amount	Calories
Mood: _______________	Energy: _______________	Total Calories: _______________		

LUNCH				
Food		Time	Amount	Calories
Mood: _______________	Energy: _______________	Total Calories: _______________		

DINNER				
Food		Time	Amount	Calories
Mood: _______________	Energy: _______________	Total Calories: _______________		

<table>
<tr><td colspan="4">SNACKS</td></tr>
</table>

Food			Time	Amount	Calories

Mood: ______________________   Energy: ______________________   Total Calories: ______________________

<table>
<tr><td>INFUSED WATER</td></tr>
</table>

Ingredients	Time	Amount	Mood After

<table>
<tr><td>EXERCISE</td></tr>
</table>

Activity	Time	Amount	Mood After

<table>
<tr><td>NOTES</td></tr>
</table>

DATE: _______________________________   WEIGHT: _______________________________

WATER INTAKE: _____________________   INFUSED WATER: _____________________

DAILY GOAL: ____

Increase Immunity   Increase Energy   Detoxification   Increase Metabolism

BREAKFAST

Food	Time	Amount	Calories

Mood: _________________   Energy: _________________   Total Calories: _________________

LUNCH

Food	Time	Amount	Calories

Mood: _________________   Energy: _________________   Total Calories: _________________

DINNER

Food	Time	Amount	Calories

Mood: _________________   Energy: _________________   Total Calories: _________________

SNACKS

Food	Time	Amount	Calories

Mood: _________________ Energy: _________________ Total Calories: _________________

INFUSED WATER

Ingredients	Time	Amount	Mood After

EXERCISE

Activity	Time	Amount	Mood After

NOTES

DATE: _______________________   WEIGHT: _______________________

WATER INTAKE: _______________   INFUSED WATER: _______________

DAILY GOAL: ____

Increase Immunity   Increase Energy   Detoxification   Increase Metabolism

BREAKFAST

Food	Time	Amount	Calories

Mood: _________________   Energy: _________________   Total Calories: _________________

LUNCH

Food	Time	Amount	Calories

Mood: _________________   Energy: _________________   Total Calories: _________________

DINNER

Food	Time	Amount	Calories

Mood: _________________   Energy: _________________   Total Calories: _________________

SNACKS			
Food	Time	Amount	Calories

Mood: _________________ Energy: _________________ Total Calories: _________________

INFUSED WATER			
Ingredients	Time	Amount	Mood After

EXERCISE			
Activity	Time	Amount	Mood After

NOTES

DATE: _________________________   WEIGHT: _________________________

WATER INTAKE: _________________________   INFUSED WATER: _________________________

DAILY GOAL: ____

Increase Immunity   Increase Energy   Detoxification   Increase Metabolism

BREAKFAST

Food	Time	Amount	Calories

Mood: _________________   Energy: _________________   Total Calories: _________________

LUNCH

Food	Time	Amount	Calories

Mood: _________________   Energy: _________________   Total Calories: _________________

DINNER

Food	Time	Amount	Calories

Mood: _________________   Energy: _________________   Total Calories: _________________

SNACKS

Food	Time	Amount	Calories

Mood: ________________   Energy: ________________   Total Calories: ________________

INFUSED WATER

Ingredients	Time	Amount	Mood After

EXERCISE

Activity	Time	Amount	Mood After

NOTES

DATE: _______________________ WEIGHT: _______________________

WATER INTAKE: _______________ INFUSED WATER: _______________

DAILY GOAL: ____

Increase Immunity   Increase Energy   Detoxification   Increase Metabolism

BREAKFAST

Food	Time	Amount	Calories

Mood: _______________ Energy: _______________ Total Calories: _______________

LUNCH

Food	Time	Amount	Calories

Mood: _______________ Energy: _______________ Total Calories: _______________

DINNER

Food	Time	Amount	Calories

Mood: _______________ Energy: _______________ Total Calories: _______________

SNACKS

Food	Time	Amount	Calories

Mood: _____________________ Energy: _____________________ Total Calories: _____________________

INFUSED WATER

Ingredients	Time	Amount	Mood After

EXERCISE

Activity	Time	Amount	Mood After

NOTES

DATE: _______________________________   WEIGHT: _______________________________

WATER INTAKE: _______________________   INFUSED WATER: _______________________

DAILY GOAL: ____

Increase Immunity   Increase Energy   Detoxification   Increase Metabolism

BREAKFAST

Food	Time	Amount	Calories

Mood: _______________   Energy: _______________   Total Calories: _______________

LUNCH

Food	Time	Amount	Calories

Mood: _______________   Energy: _______________   Total Calories: _______________

DINNER

Food	Time	Amount	Calories

Mood: _______________   Energy: _______________   Total Calories: _______________

Food	Time	Amount	Calories

Mood: _________________ Energy: _________________ Total Calories: _________________

Ingredients	Time	Amount	Mood After

Activity	Time	Amount	Mood After

DATE: _________________________ WEIGHT: _________________________

WATER INTAKE: _________________ INFUSED WATER: _________________

DAILY GOAL: ____

Increase Immunity   Increase Energy   Detoxification   Increase Metabolism

BREAKFAST

Food	Time	Amount	Calories

Mood: _________________ Energy: _________________ Total Calories: _________________

LUNCH

Food	Time	Amount	Calories

Mood: _________________ Energy: _________________ Total Calories: _________________

DINNER

Food	Time	Amount	Calories

Mood: _________________ Energy: _________________ Total Calories: _________________

SNACKS

Food	Time	Amount	Calories

Mood: _____________________ Energy: _____________________ Total Calories: _____________________

INFUSED WATER

Ingredients	Time	Amount	Mood After

EXERCISE

Activity	Time	Amount	Mood After

NOTES

DATE: ___________________________   WEIGHT: ___________________________

WATER INTAKE: ___________________   INFUSED WATER: ___________________

DAILY GOAL: ____

Increase Immunity   Increase Energy   Detoxification   Increase Metabolism

BREAKFAST

Food	Time	Amount	Calories

Mood: ___________________   Energy: ___________________   Total Calories: ___________________

LUNCH

Food	Time	Amount	Calories

Mood: ___________________   Energy: ___________________   Total Calories: ___________________

DINNER

Food	Time	Amount	Calories

Mood: ___________________   Energy: ___________________   Total Calories: ___________________

SNACKS

Food	Time	Amount	Calories

Mood: _____________________ Energy: _____________________ Total Calories: _____________________

INFUSED WATER

Ingredients	Time	Amount	Mood After

EXERCISE

Activity	Time	Amount	Mood After

NOTES

DATE: _________________________ WEIGHT: _____________________

WATER INTAKE: _________________ INFUSED WATER: _______________

DAILY GOAL: ____

Increase Immunity   Increase Energy   Detoxification   Increase Metabolism

BREAKFAST

Food	Time	Amount	Calories

Mood: _________________ Energy: _________________ Total Calories: _________________

LUNCH

Food	Time	Amount	Calories

Mood: _________________ Energy: _________________ Total Calories: _________________

DINNER

Food	Time	Amount	Calories

Mood: _________________ Energy: _________________ Total Calories: _________________

SNACKS

Food	Time	Amount	Calories

Mood: _________________   Energy: _________________   Total Calories: _______________

INFUSED WATER

Ingredients	Time	Amount	Mood After

EXERCISE

Activity	Time	Amount	Mood After

NOTES

DATE: _________________________________   WEIGHT: _________________________________

WATER INTAKE: _____________________________   INFUSED WATER: _____________________________

DAILY GOAL: ____

Increase Immunity   Increase Energy   Detoxification   Increase Metabolism

BREAKFAST

Food	Time	Amount	Calories

Mood: _____________________   Energy: _____________________   Total Calories: _____________________

LUNCH

Food	Time	Amount	Calories

Mood: _____________________   Energy: _____________________   Total Calories: _____________________

DINNER

Food	Time	Amount	Calories

Mood: _____________________   Energy: _____________________   Total Calories: _____________________

Food		Time	Amount	Calories

Mood: _____________________   Energy: _____________________   Total Calories: _____________________

Ingredients	Time	Amount	Mood After

Activity	Time	Amount	Mood After

DATE: _______________________________ WEIGHT: _______________________________

WATER INTAKE: _______________________ INFUSED WATER: _______________________

DAILY GOAL: ____

Increase Immunity   Increase Energy   Detoxification   Increase Metabolism

BREAKFAST

Food	Time	Amount	Calories

Mood: _______________ Energy: _______________ Total Calories: _______________

LUNCH

Food	Time	Amount	Calories

Mood: _______________ Energy: _______________ Total Calories: _______________

DINNER

Food	Time	Amount	Calories

Mood: _______________ Energy: _______________ Total Calories: _______________

SNACKS

Food	Time	Amount	Calories

Mood: _________________   Energy: _________________   Total Calories: _________________

INFUSED WATER

Ingredients	Time	Amount	Mood After

EXERCISE

Activity	Time	Amount	Mood After

NOTES

DATE: _________________________   WEIGHT: _____________________

WATER INTAKE: _____________________   INFUSED WATER: _____________________

DAILY GOAL: ____

Increase Immunity   Increase Energy   Detoxification   Increase Metabolism

BREAKFAST

Food	Time	Amount	Calories

Mood: _________________   Energy: _________________   Total Calories: _________________

LUNCH

Food	Time	Amount	Calories

Mood: _________________   Energy: _________________   Total Calories: _________________

DINNER

Food	Time	Amount	Calories

Mood: _________________   Energy: _________________   Total Calories: _________________

Food	Time	Amount	Calories

Mood: _________________   Energy: _________________   Total Calories: _________________

Ingredients	Time	Amount	Mood After

Activity	Time	Amount	Mood After

DATE: ___________________________   WEIGHT: ___________________________

WATER INTAKE: _______________   INFUSED WATER: _______________

DAILY GOAL: ____

Increase Immunity   Increase Energy   Detoxification   Increase Metabolism

BREAKFAST

Food	Time	Amount	Calories

Mood: _________________   Energy: _________________   Total Calories: _________________

LUNCH

Food	Time	Amount	Calories

Mood: _________________   Energy: _________________   Total Calories: _________________

DINNER

Food	Time	Amount	Calories

Mood: _________________   Energy: _________________   Total Calories: _________________

SNACKS

Food	Time	Amount	Calories

Mood: _____________________ Energy: _____________________ Total Calories: _____________________

INFUSED WATER

Ingredients	Time	Amount	Mood After

EXERCISE

Activity	Time	Amount	Mood After

NOTES

DATE: _______________________________   WEIGHT: _______________________________

WATER INTAKE: _______________________   INFUSED WATER: _______________________

DAILY GOAL: ____

Increase Immunity   Increase Energy   Detoxification   Increase Metabolism

BREAKFAST

Food		Time	Amount	Calories

Mood: _______________   Energy: _______________   Total Calories: _______________

LUNCH

Food		Time	Amount	Calories

Mood: _______________   Energy: _______________   Total Calories: _______________

DINNER

Food		Time	Amount	Calories

Mood: _______________   Energy: _______________   Total Calories: _______________

SNACKS

Food	Time	Amount	Calories

Mood: _____________________ Energy: _____________________ Total Calories: _____________________

INFUSED WATER

Ingredients	Time	Amount	Mood After

EXERCISE

Activity	Time	Amount	Mood After

NOTES

DATE: _________________________   WEIGHT: _________________________

WATER INTAKE: _________________   INFUSED WATER: _________________

DAILY GOAL: ____

Increase Immunity   Increase Energy   Detoxification   Increase Metabolism

BREAKFAST

Food	Time	Amount	Calories

Mood: _________________   Energy: _________________   Total Calories: _________________

LUNCH

Food	Time	Amount	Calories

Mood: _________________   Energy: _________________   Total Calories: _________________

DINNER

Food	Time	Amount	Calories

Mood: _________________   Energy: _________________   Total Calories: _________________

Food	Time	Amount	Calories

Mood: _____________________ Energy: _____________________ Total Calories: _____________________

INFUSED WATER

Ingredients	Time	Amount	Mood After

EXERCISE

Activity	Time	Amount	Mood After

NOTES

DATE: _______________________   WEIGHT: _______________________

WATER INTAKE: _______________   INFUSED WATER: _______________

DAILY GOAL: ____

Increase Immunity   Increase Energy   Detoxification   Increase Metabolism

BREAKFAST

Food	Time	Amount	Calories

Mood: _______________ Energy: _______________ Total Calories: _______________

LUNCH

Food	Time	Amount	Calories

Mood: _______________ Energy: _______________ Total Calories: _______________

DINNER

Food	Time	Amount	Calories

Mood: _______________ Energy: _______________ Total Calories: _______________

SNACKS

Food	Time	Amount	Calories

Mood: _________________   Energy: _________________   Total Calories: _________________

INFUSED WATER

Ingredients	Time	Amount	Mood After

EXERCISE

Activity	Time	Amount	Mood After

NOTES

DATE: ___________________________ WEIGHT: ___________________________

WATER INTAKE: ___________________ INFUSED WATER: ___________________

DAILY GOAL: ____

Increase Immunity　　　Increase Energy　　　Detoxification　　　Increase Metabolism

BREAKFAST

Food	Time	Amount	Calories

Mood: _________________ Energy: _________________ Total Calories: _________________

LUNCH

Food	Time	Amount	Calories

Mood: _________________ Energy: _________________ Total Calories: _________________

DINNER

Food	Time	Amount	Calories

Mood: _________________ Energy: _________________ Total Calories: _________________

Food	Time	Amount	Calories

Mood: _________________   Energy: _________________   Total Calories: _________________

Ingredients	Time	Amount	Mood After

Activity	Time	Amount	Mood After

DATE: ___________________________________   WEIGHT: ___________________________________

WATER INTAKE: ___________________________   INFUSED WATER: ___________________________

DAILY GOAL: ____

Increase Immunity   Increase Energy   Detoxification   Increase Metabolism

BREAKFAST

Food	Time	Amount	Calories

Mood: ___________________   Energy: ___________________   Total Calories: ___________________

LUNCH

Food	Time	Amount	Calories

Mood: ___________________   Energy: ___________________   Total Calories: ___________________

DINNER

Food	Time	Amount	Calories

Mood: ___________________   Energy: ___________________   Total Calories: ___________________

DATE: _________________________________   WEIGHT: _________________________________

WATER INTAKE: _____________________   INFUSED WATER: _____________________

DAILY GOAL: ____

Increase Immunity   Increase Energy   Detoxification   Increase Metabolism

BREAKFAST

Food	Time	Amount	Calories

Mood: _______________   Energy: _______________   Total Calories: _______________

LUNCH

Food	Time	Amount	Calories

Mood: _______________   Energy: _______________   Total Calories: _______________

DINNER

Food	Time	Amount	Calories

Mood: _______________   Energy: _______________   Total Calories: _______________

Food		Time	Amount	Calories

Mood: _____________________ Energy: _____________________ Total Calories: _____________________

Ingredients	Time	Amount	Mood After

Activity	Time	Amount	Mood After

DATE: ______________________________   WEIGHT: ______________________________

WATER INTAKE: ______________________   INFUSED WATER: ______________________

DAILY GOAL: ____

Increase Immunity   Increase Energy   Detoxification   Increase Metabolism

BREAKFAST

Food	Time	Amount	Calories

Mood: ______________   Energy: ______________   Total Calories: ______________

LUNCH

Food	Time	Amount	Calories

Mood: ______________   Energy: ______________   Total Calories: ______________

DINNER

Food	Time	Amount	Calories

Mood: ______________   Energy: ______________   Total Calories: ______________

SNACKS

Food	Time	Amount	Calories

Mood: _____________________ Energy: _____________________ Total Calories: _____________________

INFUSED WATER

Ingredients	Time	Amount	Mood After

EXERCISE

Activity	Time	Amount	Mood After

NOTES

DATE: _________________________ WEIGHT: ___________________________

WATER INTAKE: _____________________ INFUSED WATER: ___________________

DAILY GOAL: ____

Increase Immunity   Increase Energy   Detoxification   Increase Metabolism

BREAKFAST

Food	Time	Amount	Calories

Mood: _________________ Energy: _________________ Total Calories: _________________

LUNCH

Food	Time	Amount	Calories

Mood: _________________ Energy: _________________ Total Calories: _________________

DINNER

Food	Time	Amount	Calories

Mood: _________________ Energy: _________________ Total Calories: _________________

Food	Time	Amount	Calories

Mood: ______________________ | Energy: ______________________ | Total Calories: ______________________

Ingredients	Time	Amount	Mood After

Activity	Time	Amount	Mood After

DATE: _______________________________   WEIGHT: _______________________________

WATER INTAKE: _______________________   INFUSED WATER: _______________________

DAILY GOAL: ____

Increase Immunity   Increase Energy   Detoxification   Increase Metabolism

BREAKFAST

Food	Time	Amount	Calories

Mood: _______________   Energy: _______________   Total Calories: _______________

LUNCH

Food	Time	Amount	Calories

Mood: _______________   Energy: _______________   Total Calories: _______________

DINNER

Food	Time	Amount	Calories

Mood: _______________   Energy: _______________   Total Calories: _______________

Food	Time	Amount	Calories

Mood: ___________________   Energy: ___________________   Total Calories: ___________________

Ingredients	Time	Amount	Mood After

Activity	Time	Amount	Mood After

DATE: _______________________________   WEIGHT: _______________________________

WATER INTAKE: _____________________   INFUSED WATER: __________________

DAILY GOAL: ____

Increase Immunity   Increase Energy   Detoxification   Increase Metabolism

BREAKFAST

Food	Time	Amount	Calories

Mood: _______________   Energy: _______________   Total Calories: _______________

LUNCH

Food	Time	Amount	Calories

Mood: _______________   Energy: _______________   Total Calories: _______________

DINNER

Food	Time	Amount	Calories

Mood: _______________   Energy: _______________   Total Calories: _______________

Food	Time	Amount	Calories

Mood: _____________________ Energy: _____________________ Total Calories: _____________________

INFUSED WATER

Ingredients	Time	Amount	Mood After

EXERCISE

Activity	Time	Amount	Mood After

NOTES

DATE: _________________________________ WEIGHT: _________________________________

WATER INTAKE: _____________________ INFUSED WATER: _____________________

DAILY GOAL: ____

Increase Immunity   Increase Energy   Detoxification   Increase Metabolism

BREAKFAST

Food	Time	Amount	Calories

Mood: _________________ Energy: _________________ Total Calories: _________________

LUNCH

Food	Time	Amount	Calories

Mood: _________________ Energy: _________________ Total Calories: _________________

DINNER

Food	Time	Amount	Calories

Mood: _________________ Energy: _________________ Total Calories: _________________

Food	Time	Amount	Calories

Mood: _________________ Energy: _________________ Total Calories: _________________

INFUSED WATER

Ingredients	Time	Amount	Mood After

EXERCISE

Activity	Time	Amount	Mood After

NOTES

DATE: _________________________ WEIGHT: _____________________

WATER INTAKE: _______________ INFUSED WATER: _______________

DAILY GOAL: ____

Increase Immunity   Increase Energy   Detoxification   Increase Metabolism

BREAKFAST

Food	Time	Amount	Calories

Mood: _________________ Energy: _________________ Total Calories: _______________

LUNCH

Food	Time	Amount	Calories

Mood: _________________ Energy: _________________ Total Calories: _______________

DINNER

Food	Time	Amount	Calories

Mood: _________________ Energy: _________________ Total Calories: _______________

SNACKS

Food	Time	Amount	Calories

Mood: _____________________ Energy: _____________________ Total Calories: _____________________

INFUSED WATER

Ingredients	Time	Amount	Mood After

EXERCISE

Activity	Time	Amount	Mood After

NOTES

DATE: ________________________________   WEIGHT: ________________________________

WATER INTAKE: ____________________   INFUSED WATER: ____________________

DAILY GOAL: ____

Increase Immunity   Increase Energy   Detoxification   Increase Metabolism

BREAKFAST

Food		Time	Amount	Calories

Mood: ____________________   Energy: ____________________   Total Calories: ____________________

LUNCH

Food		Time	Amount	Calories

Mood: ____________________   Energy: ____________________   Total Calories: ____________________

DINNER

Food		Time	Amount	Calories

Mood: ____________________   Energy: ____________________   Total Calories: ____________________

Food	Time	Amount	Calories

Mood: ______________________ Energy: ______________________ Total Calories: ______________________

Ingredients	Time	Amount	Mood After

Activity	Time	Amount	Mood After

